# Low Carb Diet

# For Beginners

**The Ultimate Beginner's Guide To Low-Carb Diet - What to Eat and Avoid, Meal Plan & Food List, Health Benefits and Risks + 50 Proven Fat Burn Low Carb Weight Loss Recipes**

By *Isabella Evelyn*

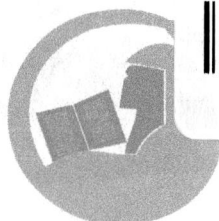

I0135247

**EFFINGO**
Publishing

For more great books visit:

**EffingoPublishing.com**

# Download another book for Free

We want to thank you for purchasing this book and offer you another book (just as long and valuable as this book), "Health & Fitness Mistakes You Don't Know You're Making", completely free.

Visit the link below to signup and receive it:

www.effingopublishing.com/gift

In this book, we will break down the most common health & fitness mistakes, you are probably committing right now, and will reveal how you can easily get in the best shape of your life!

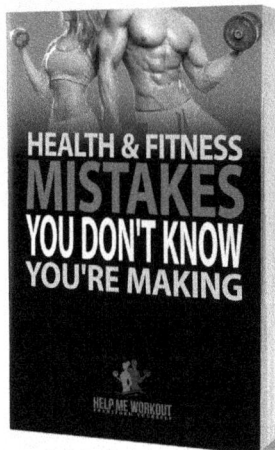

In addition to this valuable gift, you will also have an opportunity to get our new books for free, enter giveaways, and receive other valuable emails from us. Again, visit the link to sign up:

www.effingopublishing.com/gift

# TABLE OF CONTENTS

# INTRODUCTION

Many people fail in their attempts to lose weight, and it leads them to become depressed and lose motivation to try again. Many people are on a constant yo-yo weight loss cycle and want to get off that roller coaster ride. They want to be successful, yet they just can't pinpoint exactly how. If this is how you feel, you are most definitely not alone. There are many reasons that one may decide to try a low-carb diet. One of the biggest reasons is the fact that they are so effective. In general, one can lose more weight than regular diets at a significant rate of approximately two to three times a week as compared to someone who is doing a regular low-fat diet. They also are known to be safer, although we will address the health risks later on. Unfortunately, nothing in life is without some kind of risk. Some great things you will begin to notice are your blood sugar begins to stabilize. You begin to have more energy and become more cognitively alert. Low carb diets also assist considerably with food cravings as you are eating high fat and high-protein foods.

Also, before you get started, I recommend you **joining our email newsletter** to receive updates on any upcoming new book releases or promotions. You can sign-up for free, and as a bonus, you will receive a free gift. Our *"Health & Fitness Mistakes You Don't Know You're Making"* book! This book has been written to demystify, expose the top do's and don'ts and to finally equip you with the information you need to get in the best shape of your life. Due to the overwhelming amount of mis-information and lies told by magazines and self-proclaimed "gurus", it's becoming harder and harder to get reliable information to get in shape. As opposed to having to go through dozens of biased, unreliable and un-trustworthy sources to get your health & fitness information. Everything you need to help you has been broken down in this book for you to easily follow and to immediately get results to achieve your desired fitness goals in the shortest amount of time.

Once again, to join our free email newsletter and to receive a free copy of this valuable book, please visit the link and signup now: **www.effingopublishing.com/gift**

# CHAPTER 1: WHY WE DECIDE TO DIET IN THE FIRST PLACE?

Most of us have tried some strict diet at least once in their lifetime. They are not usually fun and not often because we are excited to do it. We, for some reason or another, have to change our eating patterns. There are many reasons that one may decide to try a more complex diet than a simpler one like just cutting down on calories and or fat. These days there are so many different ways to lose weight as the science behind body chemistry is continuously evolving, and we learn new things about our chemical makeup each day. Sometimes someone will experiment with various dieting techniques based on the advice of a doctor for medical reasons. Other times they do it to look sexier and enjoy the enticing cosmetic benefits that go along with it. One could be going through a rough breakup or divorce and feel the need to change their appearance to gain self-confidence back in their lives. For most people, it is a combination of a few different reasons.

# Why We Don't Always Succeed on a Diet

Diets can be confusing. What to eat when? They are also a significant addition to some people already very tight budgets. The facts are simple. Unhealthy foods are cheaper than making wholesome meals at home that require many ingredients. When you go to the grocery store, put the food away, and store the food in a secure location like a refrigerator or a freezer. Then you have to take the ingredients back out when you want to cook, then follow the recipe very carefully, which can be difficult for some people.

## Convenience Factors

We also enjoy convenience. When a fast-food joint is on the way home from work and has a drive-through menu, and you're exhausted from a long gruelling day at the office, cooking sounds like an absolute nightmare. It's hard to cook when you are tired at times. It can also be complicated to follow the strict adherence necessary to a specified chosen diet to be successful in losing weight.

## Exhaustion and Other Failure Rate Factors

Cutting a lot of calories also makes you feel more tired. With a diet, usually comes exercise. To lift weights, do cardio, and long walks, you require a lot of energy to succeed. Food is energy, and the less food we eat, the less energy we have to do the things we need to do in our lives. When we are on a diet that lowers our energy levels, how can you be successful? Another issue is that they can leave you feeling hungry and dissatisfied. When you aren't getting enough fats and proteins, you can feel tired. Do you ever notice how energetic you feel after a steak and vegetable meal? You think that way because you are eating foods that are unprocessed and not full of preservatives and sugar. This diet asks you to begin to eat more organic food, which can be quite expensive. Organic is always healthier but not required if you cannot afford it. Don't let this be a barrier, though, understand that it's possible to spend enough to satisfy your diet without breaking the bank, it just requires a little more financial budgeting and utilizing local discount food chains and coupon clipping. You can also get apps like Ibotta that pay you for your receipts.

# Chapter 2: Understanding different terms for Low Carb Diet

It is close to our natural style of eating, which is a Ketogenic-style diet. This is another way to say a low carb diet is calling it a ketogenic diet. We will use these words interchangeably so you understand that you can also find additional recipes using both terms. Many people fail in their attempts to lose weight, and it leads them to become depressed and lose motivation to try again. Many people are on a constant yo-yo weight loss cycle and want to get off that roller coaster ride. They want to be successful, yet they can't pinpoint exactly how. If this is how you feel, you are most definitely not alone.

## Explaining a Low Carb Diet and whether it is a Good Choice for You.

This book is going to give you the best possible to guide you on how to successfully implement a low-carb or ketogenic diet into your daily routine in the most simplified way possible. In the most simplified way to describe it, you stay away from pasta, sugar ridden foods, and regular bread, including both white and wheat bread. The idea is to eat more pure foods that are more natural. This can significantly change your life and energy levels. Dieters all have different goals and possible sub-goals. There are various factors that motivate different people.

- Some individuals want to lose weight because their body mass index is too high, and they want to lower their BMI.
- You may be getting older, and your metabolism is changing and slowing down, and you want to speed it back up.
- You are going to a big event and want to wear an outfit that doesn't fit quite yet.
- Your partner has asked you to lose weight.
- You have diabetes and need to change eating

- You have a bladder condition, and certain foods can irritate the lining of the bladder.

- You are having trouble getting around quickly enough because the extra weight makes it harder to breathe.

- Being over the recommended weight for your height and body style can cause back and other health issues.

It can be challenging to pick the right diet for you. It is a very frustrating decision with all the choices that you have these days. It takes much thought, consideration of your lifestyle, and budget constraints to decide on the best meal plan for you.

## Considering Your Health Issues

You have to consider other health issues that you may have and choose the diet that best fits your personalized needs as a person. What may work for someone you know, may not work at all for you. This is because we all have unique body styles and metabolic systems. Some of us burn fat quite quickly, while others have an extremely slow metabolism that makes it difficult to lose weight. Having a possible thyroid condition will also change what kind of diet, you can be on and how fast you lose the weight. It is imperative to speak to a health professional qualified in customized menus to make sure you are choosing the safest diet as well as most effective for you.

# We All Feel Unsure of Which Diet to Choose

If you are feeling unsure of what type of diet to go for, you're not alone on that either. Many individuals are not successful from a conventional diet, and they fail because they are feeling dissatisfied and partially starved. If you are constantly craving food and always hungry, how are you supposed to meet your weight loss goals? Most diets require an extreme amount of discipline and strict workout schedules. A useful aspect of a low carb diet, however, gives an individual enough protein and fat to keep their motivation up and continue with the diet. It has years of research and success stories, backing it's incredibly high success rate for many. That's why it continues to be extremely popular, while other diet fads tend to come and go. A low carb or ketogenic diet is usually an excellent choice for most people, but again consult an expert and physician before starting any diet. This is to be entirely sure if it's the right diet for your personalized health needs and will not harm your health.

## Explaining the Diet in Detail

You may be confused with if you should go completely fat-free or low-fat, try Slim Fast, or complete fasting. There are so many fad diets that work for some and fail for others. The goal of this book is going to explain to you how to be a success story on a low carb or ketogenic diet and other factors that will influence your decision if this is the right diet for you.

# Chapter 3: Why Go on a Low Carb Diet, What to Expect and How Does it Work Exactly?

There are many reasons that one may decide to try a low-carb diet. One of the biggest reasons is the fact that they are so useful. In general, one can lose more weight than regular diets at a significant rate of approximately two to three times a week as compared to someone who is doing a proper low-fat diet. They also are known to be safer, although we will address the health risks later on. Unfortunately, nothing in life is without some risk. Some great things you will begin to notice are your blood sugar begins to stabilize. You begin to have more energy and become more cognitively alert. Low carb diets also assist considerably with food cravings as you are eating high fat and high-protein foods. These types of meals are great because they tend to satisfy a human being without desires for more extended periods. You stop focusing on lower calorie and lower fat foods and focus on low carb, high fat, high-protein foods. These diets create chemistry in your body that makes you feel fuller. When you are not hungry, you end up eating a lot less and feel a lot more energetic naturally. Those sugary food cravings begin to decrease because you are stabilizing your cravings naturally by changing your diet. This helps one to stay on a diet longer because hunger pains are not occurring nearly as much as traditional diets.

## How Many Carbs Can You Eat?

A low carb diet has no set number of carbs. To be considered a low-carbohydrate diet, you focus on eating proteins and fats that are on the lower end of the spectrum from anywhere from twenty to two hundred carbs per day. Some low carb diets are more lenient and allow for more carbohydrates, while more strict ketogenic diets offer less. You can still eat many foods that you enjoy. You are just cutting out a lot of overly processed foods, starches, and bread-type products. There are a lot of things that you can still enjoy. We will show you in the recipe section how to make your diet easier to follow and less complex to understand. You will begin to eat more natural foods geared towards losing weight long term in the human body, instead of types of foods comprised of overly processed and chemically enhanced choices. It is closer to what our ancestors would eat on a deficient carb diet or ketogenic diet. Another great thing is the ability to still eat at all your favorite restaurants. You ask the server to hold the bread if it is offered. You most definitely can enjoy as much meat as you like, leaving you more energetic and satisfied.

# Explaining the Distinct Difference Between Good and Bad Carbs

After reading the above information, you may think that all carbs are bad, but it's not as cut and dry and that. There are two types of carbohydrates. Some are good, and some are bad carbs. In vegetables and fruits, there are carbohydrates, known as good carbs. It is because they are occurring in naturally grown foods. Fiber is something that we need to keep our digestive systems on the right track. A good carbohydrate contains a high amount of fiber, as well. You need to keep track of making sure you are under the recommended amount of grams a day of carbohydrates of 200 on the higher end of the spectrum and 20 on the lower end.

## Generalized Good Ketogenic Diet Foods

Our recipes will explain many of the foods that you can have while ingesting a low-carbohydrate diet.

- Veggies and fruits are naturally high in fiber, but you want to moderate any fruits and vegetables that contain high levels of carbs. You are allowed them; however, in the diet, pay attention to the number of carbs in each fruit and vegetable that you put in your body. This also keeps your blood sugar levels from spiking dramatically.
- When choosing meats, try to pick organic grass-fed meats.

- Wild-caught fish is also a great choice, if you cannot access wild-caught fish, then read the label and see how much processing has been done to it and avoid highly processed fish. Always be careful to mix in enough fish into your diet to be healthy, but not too much as fish contains a small amount of mercury.
- Greek Yogurt can also be considered a great choice.
- You can have some nuts and legumes.
- You can even have dark chocolate in moderation as long as it has a minimum of seventy percent cocoa.
- Fruits are always in moderation, as explained earlier because some are high in carbs but don't cut them out completely. Just have self-control.
- You can have butter and olive oil to use for cooking and flavor, as well as coconut oil.
- Coffee is still okay to consume as long as you are not adding sugar to it. The same principle goes with tea, as well.
- Eggs are an essential part of the diet and contain high levels of protein.
- Peanut butter is excellent, as well.

- There is a vast selection of cheeses that you can have.

# Follow A Professionals Advice

When looking at carbohydrates that are considered bad, you want to look into foods that most of the nutrients and naturally occurring fibres are taken away during processing. Go for lower sugar fruits rather than higher sugar ones. You can have legumes, as stated above, but in moderation. You want to keep to the 20 grams to 200 grams of carbs a day range that has been recommended by a professional dietician or physician. Some of us can handle a very low carb plan, while others cannot go too low. What one person can handle in cutting down on carbohydrates, another may not be able to. There is no technical number for what is considered a low carb plan. At its simplest, you are lowering the carbs from what you usually have been eating to an amount that you can handle. Some can handle the lower end of the spectrum and can do 20-60 grams of carbs a day without an issue. Others need anywhere from 100 to 200 grams. This is still considered a moderately low carb ketogenic diet.

# Foods You Definitely Want to Avoid Eating

Avoid anything with added sugars like cereals, as well as white or bleached grains and bread. Glucose levels rise when sugars and grains are refined. Stay away from high fructose corn syrup and just essential low-fat foods that do not consider carbohydrate levels. You'll want to eliminate any boxed foods from your home that could contain preservatives. Examples of these foods could be frozen pizzas, ice creams, and shakes. This may be difficult at; first, you're going to have to make some problematic meal decisions. More foods to avoid-

- Highly processed soda and soft drinks
- Candy as it is high in sugar

- No vegetable oils

- No trans fats

- Stay away from pasta and bread as much as possible even if they contain the good carbs because, in a serving of pasta, you are ingesting approximately 25 grams of carbohydrates.

- Artificial sweetening items are also a no-no, such as

- packaged snacks like sweets that are highly processed and potato chips.

- Cereals that you would eat for breakfast as they have more than fifty carbs per serving.

- Oats have approximately 66 grams of carbohydrates, meaning you are going over your daily limit with one serving of them if on the low end 20-60 carb a day diet.

- Bananas are a fruit to limit because it is a natural food, but there are better carbs to ingest as this high-sugar food contains 23 grams of carbs.

- Beans may be high in nutritional value but are not precisely ideal for a lower-carb diet plan.

- Potatoes and yams are very high carb foods.

- Cranberries are full of sugars.

- Tropical fruits have more sugar than other types of fruits. Pineapples and mangos also contain high levels of carbs.

- As mentioned before, white bread is not right on this diet, but neither is brown bread. A piece here and there is fine but proceed with extreme caution and keep track of your daily carb intake if you slip up and eat some bread.

## Possible Medical Benefits

Some individuals are put on a low-carb diet by their doctor to benefit them health-wise. A great benefit is this kind of diet trigger higher levels of HDL Cholesterol, which is known as the healthier type of cholesterol. There is also a wrong type of cholesterol known as LDL. Lowering the intake of the wrong kind will considerably reduce your risk of heart disease. The low carb diet works much better than a low-fat diet to put your cholesterol levels in both categories in the proper level range. Here are some more benefits to going on a low carb diet-

- There is something known as triglycerides that are floating around in the body. These are the types of fat molecules that move around in the bloodstream.
- Having a high level of them will possibly perpetuate a stronger chance of heart issues as you age.
- When you make a conscious choice to remove them from your diet deliberately, these are significantly reduced. Low-fat diets cause triglycerides to rise.
- As a general rule, the entire reason for changing your diet is to lose fat and gain muscle. Strangely enough, low-fat diets have the opposite reaction.
- A significant percent body fat that you lose on a diet that is lower in carbohydrates comes from the stomach area as well as the liver.
- There are two significant kinds of fat. One is known as subcutaneous fat, while the other is known as visceral fat. The difference between the two is that visceral fat is located in the stomach area or cavity,

while subcutaneous fat is the fat found beneath your skin.

- One of the best perks of this diet is a weight loss in the abdominal cavity.
- If you accumulate too much visceral fat that surrounds the areas, your crucial organs can cause them to become majorly inflamed.
- This also includes your liver, which, when inflamed, can cause significant damage.
- Utilizing a low carb diet lifestyle also promotes higher metabolic functioning.
- Losing belly fat is the hardest part of a weight-loss journey for many individuals. This diet decreases your belly fat loss significantly, giving you the confidence to keep going instead of giving up as most people do on traditional diets.
- Going on a carefully measured low carb diet will reduce the amount of sugar in your blood, and natural insulin levels will be reduced.
- Diabetic individuals tend to build resistance to insulin after a while, and changing diet can help to

keep medications for diabetes working correctly if you are taking care of your food intake.

- It is possible to even cut down drastically on insulin shots and the dosages needed by up to fifty percent.

- You always want to get medical advice; however, from a professional dietician or doctor before going on a diet, whether you are considered healthy or have diabetes as changing a diet drastically always requires medical approval.

- Because your blood pressure is lowered, you can avoid many health issues in the future.

- Having lowered blood pressure can eradicate several health issues such as heart problems, future strokes, and kidney issues, which can turn into kidney failure. If you cut carbs, you are significantly lowering your blood pressure and your risk of these diseases.

- A health problem known as metabolic syndrome is known to be associated with other diets and uncontrolled eating, thus increasing your risk of diabetes and heart disease. Metabolic syndrome has similar symptoms of stomach obesity, heightened blood pressure and blood sugar, high triglycerides, and low "good" HDL levels.

- We have discussed the benefits that cutting carbs has on your HDL or good cholesterol. We haven't talked much about what a low carb diet does for your LDL or bad cholesterol. Those with high LDL have a much-enhanced chance of having a single heart attack or multiple heart attacks.

- The size of a person's LDL particles is a large part of their risk factors that contribute to having heart attacks.

- The smaller the particles are, the higher the risk of a major heart attack.

- On the flip side, the larger the LDL particles are, the lower your risk is for having an unexpected heart attack.

- A low carb intake will make the size of your LDL particles larger and lower your heart disease risks.

- Our brains need some glucose to function effectively, so be aware of your intake and make sure you have enough.

- Some parts of the brain can only function when this is present—low carb diet help to keep the proper levels of glucose that need to be stabilized.

- Another area of the brain, which is quite large, also burns ketones, which are created during starvation or when you reduce your carb intake below the low end of the spectrum of 20 grams of carbs.

- The ketogenic diet has been used for years to prevent epileptic seizures in those individuals who don't respond well to typical drug regimens.

- Low carb diets and ketogenic diets are continuously being studied to check the health benefits associated with other disorders like those who have Alzheimer's and Parkinson's disease.

- There are debating ideas on what these diets do to the body to cause such dramatic weight loss results, but evidence keeps showing up that they do work exceedingly well.

- When you restrict your carbohydrates, it lowers insulin levels. This is what regulates how much energy we have to be active in our daily lives and influences the blood sugar levels in our body. Insulin is what tells our cells that produce fat when to store it and when to let it go.

- On a low carb diet, insulin gets a signal inside the body to take blood sugar from the bloodstream and burn that instead of the fat we want to get rid of.
- Insulin impacts a process in the body called lipogenesis or the creation of fat and can also stimulate lipolysis, which is how we burn fat. It helps in both areas, thus causing more dramatic weight loss results than a low calorie or low-fat diet alone.
- Restricting carbohydrates makes it, so the fat isn't stuck in the fat cells, and the body can then use it to produce higher amounts of energy to get through the day, which in turn leads to fewer cravings for food.

# Lose Water Weight Early on in the Diet

There have been numerous studies done on the effectiveness of a low-carbohydrate meal plan. It was a massive fad for years to eat low carb diets and continues to gain popularity with those looking to reap the benefits of said diet. Losing water weight early on is a major benefit of ketogenic eating. This also helps to keep you motivated because you see instantaneous results on the scale. Some studies indicate that the low carb diet plans are the most effective during the first half a year of a diet than traditional diet plans. Human beings like to see fast and attainable results. We tend to be impatient creatures. If we don't see some results quickly, or as expected in mind, we tend to give up.

# Keeping the Motivation Up

Losing water weight gives us the motivation that we need to keep on going to lose the fat that they desire to lose. In fact, during the very beginning of a low carb weight loss journey, during the first week or two, people tend to drop weight exceedingly fast, which gives them the much-needed motivation to keep going on the low-carb diet. It is a two-part process that causes water weight to be lost so quickly. When you stop eating so many carbohydrates, the glycogen levels inside your body decrease, and this binds to water. When the diet begins, the extra water that has been holding on goes along with it. It also involves insulin again. When your insulin levels drop, your kidneys start to get rid of the salt that has accumulated in the body, which causes bloating. Our bodies store carbohydrates in the form of glycogen, which attaches to our muscles, and when we start to cut down and carbs, the glycogen levels naturally go down as well, and the water weight with it. On a regular diet, this does not happen nearly as quickly, causing people to feel like the diet is not working, and they lose motivation and go back to their old eating patterns. It doesn't matter whether the calories on a regular diet are dropped to a considerable degree; The water weight loss is not nearly the same as it is on a low-carb diet.

# Chapter 4: Must know risks of a Low Carbohydrate Diet

In great length, we thoroughly discussed all the benefits of a low carb diet. There are two sides to every coin, and you need to be made aware that there are risks associated with ketogenic and low carb diets. If you're going to focus on the good aspects of low carb intake, you have to talk about the bad factors in such a drastic change in living.

- The very first risk on our list is critically necessary for proper liver functioning. Our liver stores carbohydrates in the form of the compound known as glycogen, which stores glucose.

- The disadvantage of low carb consumption in highly active people is that you can easily burn through 600 calories in a day with this diet. 600 is the base amount of calories needed to survive for the average human daily without suffering too many consequences. When you are burning calories at that high level of a frantic pace, many of you will want to make sure you don't eliminate carbs if heavily active.

- If you're not careful with your carb intake on the low consumption end, you may have to stop too high-intensity workouts.
- This means limited weight training, and you deny yourself the ability to gain lean muscle and increase your metabolism.
- High cholesterol is a significant risk of low carb diets that may consist of too much fatty protein. It is recommended that with a low carb diet, you ingest higher levels of protein daily.
- However, like anything with dieting, it's about the amount you eat. The low carb/ ketogenic diet plan is designed to target hunger and causes you to have less of it.
- As with anything, balance is key. It's essential to eat protein in a balanced amount. Don't try only to eat chicken breast every night. Mix it up with steak, fish, and other proteins.

- If you're a person with kidney problems, be careful once again with your protein intake while on this diet, too much of it can worsen your health.

- The conditions that can result from a low carb diet are osteoporosis and kidney stones. Both can result from higher than normal levels of protein.

- The amount of calcium in the urine can also rise if you're not careful. This is one of the most significant and most critical factors that may cause a potential kidney stone.

- The importance of monitoring your diet is so critical, many of you need to make sure you have enough carbs, not too many, and not too little.

- If you are not careful with having enough vegetables, you can decrease your fiber intake because of the lack of some plant type foods, which could increase the possible risk factors of digestive types of cancers and cardiovascular disease.

- Another issue could also be constipation and bowel issues. Speak honestly and frankly with your primary doctor if any of these symptoms begin to occur.

- Start with a list of questions you wish to ask and also ask about what types of foods you can eat while maintaining your diet.

- Too little fruit can lead to a lack of vitamin C and potassium. These are known as your phytonutrient and antioxidants.

- These are two substances believed to be very beneficial to the human body and are used to prevent damaging agents from harming the body by ridding from the system. Antioxidants are also proven to help prevent a variety of cancers.

# CHAPTER 5: HELPFUL TIPS FOR COOKING AND MEAL PREPARATION

Eating low-carb, high-fat includes getting back to wholesome, real, unprocessed food. Some have even called it vintage eating. If you like to cook, you'll find delicious meals below to make for breakfast, lunch, and dinner.

# Diet Tips and Tricks That You Can Try

Depending on the person, some can skip breakfast and stick with coffee and milk if you're not starving. Generally, after about a week of doing a low-carb high-fat diet, the hunger pains that they were experiencing, start to disappear. This is why it is much easier to skip a meal here and there. Also, when you skip a meal, you save money and possibly make your diet more effective because you are eating less. Skipping meals here and there is known as intermittent fasting, and you can do it on a low-carb diet. It is just skipping meals here and there, and when you are on the low carb diet, you feel fuller all the time. A great trick to use is to make more servings at once. When you have a busy day coming up, the day before making yourself two meals instead of one, so you don't have to worry about cooking when you have no time in your schedule.

## Freezing Your Food and Other Tricks

Another great tip is always to freeze what you don't eat right away. Eating foods like low carb casseroles, beef stroganoff, and foods that are easily freezable, you can warm up quickly and effectively. So many low-carb recipes are easily able to be frozen and taste just as high when you reheat it. Another benefit of a low-carb diet is that you can repeat what you like that is low carb as often as you want. If you wish to eat eggs every day, go ahead. If you're going to have a steak a couple of times a week, you can do that as well. There are so many low-carb recipes that you can repeatedly make and still lose weight. There's also making up no-cook plates for yourself.

Having sliced meat from the deli and your favorite kind of cheese available is a great way not to have to cook. Vegetables are also something that you can always snack on whenever you want. If you really want something that will last for a while, boil up some eggs and have them for a few days. You can also make a vegetable dip up in advance and use that to make your veggies taste more delicious.

## Drink Plenty of Water

It is critical when you are on a low-carb diet, to make sure you are not skipping drinking water and decreasing your generalized liquid intake. Sparkling water is something that you can have an unlimited amount of on a ketogenic diet. Drinking water also makes you feel less hungry, the more water you drink, the less hungry you are going to feel.

# Chapter 6: 50 Easy Recipes to Follow and Various Meals to Make a Complete Low Carb Diet including snacks and full meals and Deserts

## 1.Delicious Low Carb Breakfast Pizza

Pizza is no longer just for lunch and dinner; it is also a tasty breakfast treat. Enjoy this recipe that you can modify the toppings to your liking.

**Crust ingredients**

- ½ cup protein powder with half cup whey isolate that is not flavored
- Half a teaspoon of regular baking powder
- Half tsp garlic of the granulated variety
- half tsp regular table salt
- Half tsp seasoning that is Italian mix

- 3 ounces of Parmesan cheese that is finely grated
- 3 ounces of chopped mozzarella cheese
- Two ounces of cream cheese
- Four tablespoons of olive oil
- One to two eggs

## Pizza Toppings

- 3 ounces of plain cream cheese
- 4 tablespoons of tomato sauce that are not sweetened or unsweetened tomato sauce
- 2 eggs scrambled
- 8 ounces of beef or sausage finely ground like hamburger meat.
- Three-quarters of a cup of finely cut up bacon

- 9 ounces of packaged and pre-shredded cheddar cheese, or you can grate your own if you are using a block of cheese.

## Instructions

- Make sure to warm the oven to 375°F.

- Take the ingredients for the crust portion and put together in a bigger size bowl.

- Use parchment paper with a baking sheet or a pizza stone with parchment paper.

- Using a spatula or regular wood spoon, mix the ingredients and smooth the pizza crust into 9 inches round.

- Another option is to make miniature pizzas using cutting the dough into four sections to create four small pizzas.

- Bake the crust for approximately 8 to 12 minutes until it is a beautiful golden-brown colour.

- Take your pizza crust out of your oven

- Add the toppings from the ingredients list with the cheese being the first thing you add and then put the other toppings on top of it to create an even distribution.

- When you're done with this, put the pizza in the oven again and cook until all of the toppings are cooked evenly.

# 2. Zuppa Toscana the Low Carb Way

Ingredients required for this delicious and healthy lunch recipe-

- 7 slices of bacon cut into one-inch pieces
- One pound of sausage
- 3 garlic cloves
- One onion diced and chopped very finely
- Two 32-ounce packages of chicken broth
- One cube of chicken bouillon
- One-half cup of water, the faucet water is fine
- Chop up 5 cups of cauliflower florets
- Three and a quarter cups of chopped kale that is stemmed
- Half of a cup of half-and-half or creamer
- 5/8 cup of Parmesan cheese

**Instructions**

- Get a large pot to cook the sausage in.
- Use the medium-high setting.

- Cook for five to seven minutes.
- Keep in the pot until it's brown and can crumble easily
- Pour the grease in a drainage area that is safe
- Put the sausage on a plate to the side
- Use the same medium to high settings and cook bacon until crisp 3-5 minutes
- Put bacon to the side
- Drain it until there are 2 teaspoons left inside the pot
- Add the chopped onion and garlic in the same pot until it softens in around five to six minutes
- Next, put bacon and sausage back in the pot
- Add the water, bouillon cube and chicken broth, keep onions and garlic in the bowl
- Add pepper to your preference
- Put kale in the pan along with the half-and-half
- Simmer this for 5 minutes
- Add Parmesan cheese to taste preference
- Serve meal

# 3. Beef Stroganoff for Dinner Made Easy and Low Carb

This low carb version of classic beef stroganoff is just as delicious as the original version but leaves you feeling much fuller for more amounts of time.

140 min prep and cook time with only 30 min preparation time and one hour in the oven. This makes it a perfectly easy and freezable meal.

## Ingredients

- Use a half teaspoon of salt
- 2 lbs of beef chuck roast
- 3 sliced green onions
- 3 teaspoons black pepper
- 5 ounces of butter or margarine
- Four tablespoons flour
- Condensed can beef broth
- Prepared mustard containing one ounce

- Can of sliced mushrooms or a package of small fresh mushrooms the size of an essential can.
- Drain them if from a can
- Third of a cup white wine
- A third of a cup of sour cream
- Collect the freeze and fat from the roast and slice the meat.
- Soak up grease and fat taken from the roast and cut meat into strips of half an inch by 2.5 inches long.
- Use half a teaspoon of salt and pepper to sprinkle over the strips.

**Instructions**

- Using a large frying pan set to medium heat
- Melt butter and cook the beef strips until brown. They cook quickly so when finished, set them to the side
- Throw the onions in the pan for four to 5 mins, cooking with the beef strips at the same time.
- Take the beef broth, poor in until it boils.

- The flour needs to be stirred into the juices made by the rest of the ingredients

- Stir every thirty seconds.

- Stir in mustard and lower the heat setting

- Let it simmer for about an hour, depending on various factors of pan quality and how hot the stove is.

- Before serving, approximately five minutes before, add the white wine and sour and cream.

# 4.Amazing Berry Low Carb pancakes with Whipped Cream Breakfast Delight

If you love pancakes, you may still have them on this diet. They are just as tasty as the original batter variety.

## Ingredients

- Four eggs
- Seven ounces of plain cottage cheese
- One tablespoon of psyllium husk powder that is ground
- Two ounces of coconut oil or regular butter or margarine
- Two ounces of frozen but thawed raspberries or fresh ones are best
- You can also substitute blueberries or strawberries for raspberries
- One cup of the heavy-style whip cream

## Instructions

• Combine the cottage cheese eggs, and psyllium husk in a bowl stirring until thoroughly mixed.

• Leave alone for four to five minutes to allow it to become thick.

• Get a nonstick skillet and heat it with oil from coconuts or the margarine or butter. Once it is ready, you can go to the next step.

• Heat up the pancakes using the medium setting for approximately three to five minutes on one side, then flip over. Keep size in mind as too large makes them difficult to turn over.

• Put the cream in a different bowl and stir it up

• Choose the type of berries that you want and add whipped cream

• Serve on a plate

# 5.Steak Chili Delight

If you are a chili lover, this recipe is for you. It is detailed and tasty with the major food health groups included. You may substitute any vegetables with ones that you may prefer instead, making it incredibly versatile.

## Ingredients

- 4 lbs one-inch steak cubes made from beef top round steak
- One-quarter cup of canola oil
- 4 garlic cloves, minced into tiny pieces
- Two and a half cups of diced onions also chopped up very small
- 2 and a half cups of water set apart separately the 2 cups from the half cup
- 2 and a quarter cups tiny pieces of chopped celery
- Three 14.5-ounce cans of undrained tomatoes
- Two cans of fifteen ounces each of salt-free tomato sauce

- One pound of salsa of your favorite variety

- Three tablespoons of powdered chili

- Two-and-a-half-teaspoon cumin ground up and dried if using out of a garden

- Two teaspoons of oregano that is dried

- One and a half teaspoons of black pepper, but this can be altered to your taste preference.

- A quarter cup of regular grocery store flour, you may also use organic if you choose to.

- A quarter cup of cornmeal that is yellow

- Additional options to add include low-fat sour cream, low-fat shredded cheese of your liking, olives, and chopped up peppers.

**Instructions**

- In a conventional oven setting on the stovetop, on medium-high temperature, cook garlic and steak until cooked thoroughly. Always keep stirring so that you have it evenly appropriately cooked.

- Add in the required amount of onions. This can also be altered if you prefer less or more onion flavor.

- Watch your food for an approximate amount of time - around five to seven minutes; make sure to keep cooking and stirring.

- Add in and mix the two cups of water along with the additional nine ingredients except for flour and cornmeal until it comes to the boiling point.

- Lower the heat to a simmer and cover for two hours approximately until it is tender and smooth to the touch and cooked well.

- Combine flour, cornmeal, and the other half of a cup of water that you were instructed to set aside in the ingredients section.

- The next step is to begin to mix it into an extremely thick and creamy texture.

- Once the chili is boiling, put in the mixture of flour and cornmeal and evenly disperse the ingredients.

- Keep cooking and stirring for approximately two to three minutes until it is quite thick.

- Next, you can add the additional ingredients mentioned at the bottom of the ingredients list, but pick whichever ones you prefer.

- This is your meal, alter it slightly as you wish.

Once done, put in bowls and serve, and you should have approximately twenty servings. They can be put in the fridge and reheated to your liking for a few more days.

# 6. Keto Steak Rolls

Enjoy this easy-to-make dinner recipe that is simple to create an easy meal

## Ingredients

- One and a half lbs of top round steak that is sliced very thin
- One half of a cup of marinade for steaks. Pick your favorite flavor or use one teaspoon of diced garlic and two tablespoons of olive oil
- one larger sized pepper that is cut into slices shaped like strips of your favorite type of either red bell peppers or green peppers.
- one cup of green beans.
- An onion that is finely chopped up

## Directions

- Place your steak in a baggie and let it soak in the marinade of your choosing for at least five minutes. The longer you wait, the better it will taste, however.

- Set your oven temp to three hundred and fifty degrees.

- Get a bigger sized frying pan. Put cooking spray or olive oil in the bottom, enough to fully cover the pan.

- Take the steak that is sliced thinly and make them into even smaller strips that are preferable to the size that you want.

- Take the steak and wrap it around your choice of peppers, onions, and green beans.

- Cook the steak in the frying pan for a minute on each side at a time. Keep on rotating until the meat is thoroughly cooked.

- Get a baking sheet and put the wrapped pieces of steak and veggies on the sheet and place in the oven that you had set to three hundred and fifty degrees.

- Cook the steak rolls for around ten to fifteen minutes until it is a beautiful brown colour.

- Serve on small dinner plates.

# 7.Low Carb Breakfast Cereal

This is a simple recipe that anyone can make. It is low carb and great for the chilly months coming up. It is versatile, like oatmeal, but a low carb version of it. You can be more daring with the ingredients like adding cinnamon or peanut butter.

## Ingredients

• Three-quarter cup of broken up hazelnuts

• Three quarter s cup almonds ground up

• Half cup flaxseed

• Half cup of oat bran

• Half cup wheat bran

• Half cup regular oatmeal (This is entirely optional and can be left out if you're on very low carb diet)

## Instructions

• Arrange all the items into a bowl. Cover and mix well as well as shake until evenly distributed.

• Cover it and put in the fridge or it will get spoiled, and it will last for approximately 90 days.

# 8.Berry Porridge

• Four tablespoons of dry oat mix

• 240 ml of natural almond milk

• 3/5 teaspoon cinnamon

• Add fruits such as apples, peaches, or berries.

**Directions**

• Using a container, start mixing the dry mix, almond milk, fruit of your choosing, and cinnamon.

• Set the microwave at one hundred percent.

• Set the timer for one to two minutes and check it every 30 seconds.

• Allow the porridge to sit and thicken naturally for 5 minutes.

• Put in a bowl and serve to guests.

# 9.Mushroom and walnut roasted with grits and cauliflower:

## Ingredients

• Five ounces of Portobello mushrooms diced to your preferred size

• Two fresh cloves of minced garlic

• Rosemary a single tablespoon

• A single tablespoon of smoked paprika

• One tablespoon of vegetable oil

• Half cup of chopped walnuts

• Medium head of cauliflower

• One cup of low-fat milk

• Half cup of water

• One cup of shredded extra sharp cheddar

• One and a half tablespoons of butter

• Add salt for extra flavor as preferred

## Instructions

• Line a baking sheet with tinfoil and heat your oven to 400 degrees Fahrenheit.

• Slowly pour your vegetable oil over your mushrooms, garlic, walnuts, smoked paprika, and rosemary, combined in a small dish.

• Make sure you mix all of these and properly spread your oil throughout the meal.

•Take your baking sheet and make sure to take your mixture and place it evenly, then wait for 14-15 minutes.

• Blend or dice your cauliflower to a very fine size.

• Heat a medium pot with a half pot of water on top. Your fine cauliflower covered for five minutes until tender and crispy.

• Mix your low-fat milk into your cauliflower grits and stir in.

• Let simmer on a low flame for 3 half mins.

• Add your butter and extra sharp cheddar and keep on low flame.

• Add your preferred amount of salt with another quarter cup of water.

• Take your baking sheet with your mushrooms cooking until a deep brown colour, and soft texture is present.

• Your meal is complete by putting the mushrooms on your cauliflower grit mix and serving.

# 10. Fresh Beets Salad and Skillet Cooked Cod.

## Ingredients

- Two pounds of fresh fillet cod
- Two and a half ounces of capers
- One and a half tablespoons of butter or margarine
- Peppercorn with salt
- Diced beets boiled

## Instructions

- Add pepper and salt to the fish you are planning to cook to the level of your liking.
- Put the fish in a frying pan with medium heat for 3 minutes on one side, flip it over and fry it another three minutes on the other side.
- In a dish, put together the caper's cubed beets, lemon juice, dill, and more salt and pepper.
- Mix it up.

- In a cooking pot, bring to a boil your cauliflower broccoli and carrots in water that is slated for approximately 5 minutes.

- Get a saucepan that has a thick bottom and heat it with medium heat.

- Next, put butter that is cut into cubes, next whisk the butter until it reaches the golden colour in the pan that you heated up.

- Turn the heat off on the butter.

- Put the card on a plate with the vegetables that you boiled and dump the butter over them. Also, put the beets next to it.

# 11. Tasty Homemade Trail Mix Snack

In general, a trail mix tends to include many high-carbohydrate tape ingredients. However, you can make a trail mix that is low carb, and this recipe will show you an easy way to make a delicious mix that you can be satisfied with.

Put together the following ingredients, and directions included

• One and a half cups of pecan

• One and a half cups of walnuts that are finely diced up

• Roast one cup of pumpkin seeds

• One cup of unsweetened coconut flakes

• Shake in a baggie and separate into individual servings

# 12. Pork and Asian veggie bowl

This exotic dish from the East orient will both delight and entice you with its variety of mouth-watering flavors. You can always substitute some of the vegetables for others that you prefer.

## Ingredients

- Three fresh green onions
- A quarter ounce of cilantro
- One clove of fresh garlic.
- A quarter ounce of ginger
- Half a serrano pepper
- Three ounces fresh or canned brown mushrooms
- 4 ounces of bok choy cabbage
- One fresh garden tomato or one small can of tomatoes
- A single cube of dehydrated Chicken stock cube
- A tablespoon of organic tamari•
- One tablespoon of extra virgin olive oil.

- 9 ounces of pork loin, tenderloin

## Instructions

• Begin by chopping your fresh green onion into small pieces.

• Pluck the stems from your fresh mushrooms.

• In quarter-inch pieces, dice your brown mushrooms, then find your cilantro and cut it into small pieces of your preference.

• You'll want to get your ginger out next and cut very fine.

• Take your mushrooms and cut into fine pieces just like your ginger, set both aside in a separate area.

• Continue by removing all of the seeds in your serrano pepper then throw it in the trash.

• Cut it up to a very fine degree and set to the side with your other ready to go ingredients and cut the end of your bok choy and slice them thin.

• Cut your tomato in half, then cut those halves into thirds and place to the side.

• After taking a paper towel to rub dry your pork tenderloin, be sure to slice into quarter-inch pieces.

• Heat a medium skillet with a tablespoon of extra virgin olive oil.

• When your pan has heated, put your tenderloin into your skillet, let cook for two and a half to three minutes until a nice crispy brown that is fully cooked on both sides.

• Remove when done and set your tenderloin to the side.

• Get yourself another pot and bring to a boil with your chicken stock, tamari sauce, and two cups of water ready to cook on high heat.

• Add your mushrooms, Serrano, garlic, ginger,

  • and your baby bok choy cabbage and simmer all of this on medium to medium high-level heat until mushrooms are soft for about four to six minutes.

  • Take your pork, tomato, and green onions, then add your cilantro and for a minute heat it up.

  • You can now turn the heat off and serve your meal to your guests or yourself.

# 13. Burger patties with tomato sauce with a side of fried cabbage

## Ingredients

• Two pounds of ground-up beef

• A single egg

• Two ounces of feta cheese that are already crumbled.

• Two and a half ounces of parsley that is preferably from a fresh garden or fresh from the store

• Two tablespoons of butter or margarine

• One tablespoon of extra virgin olive oil

## The Fried Cabbage Ingredients

• One and a half pounds of green cabbage that is shredded up finely into smaller pieces

• Five ounces of butter

• Salt and pepper to your liking

## Instructions

• Take all of your ingredients for your burgers and add hamburger to a big bowl.

• Use a large wooden spoon and blend them all together.

• Use your hands to make eight burger patties.

• Take a skillet and add butter and extra virgin olive oil.

• Put your skillet on a medium flame for ten minutes or until your burgers are nice dark brown,

• Cook both sides evenly.

• Mix tomato paste and cream in a bowl.

• Combine this mixture to the pan when your burgers are close to done.

• Let the mixture in the skillet and allow it to cook to a simmer then add your desired levels of salt and pepper.

• Add parsley on top of the meal before serving.

• Using a food processor or a sharpened knife, make sure your cabbage is shredded.

• Add butter or margarine to a skillet.

• For the cabbage portion, cook up the cabbage on a medium to medium-high heat for around sixteen minutes until your cabbage is a nice golden-brown colour on the edges.

• Mix and add butter or margarine to the cabbage.

• Let the pan simmer for a few minutes, then serve your cabbage with burgers.

# 14. Tuna salad lettuce wraps

An impressive fact about canned tuna is that it contains absolutely zero carbs and close to 20 grams of protein. It is extremely healthy to have a few times a week, but don't overdo because there is mercury in all fish.

## Ingredients

• Three ounces of a can of tuna

• A Quarter cup of mayonnaise

• A Quarter cup of celery that is diced

• Add salt and pepper to your preference either using a small amount or a larger amount sprinkle it however you like

• One larger sized piece of butter lettuce leaf

## Instructions

• Mix of your ingredients in a bowl beside the lettuce leaf.

• Take the lettuce leaf and unroll it and place the mixed tuna salad you made into the wrap.

• Spread the mix out evenly and wrap it tightly using the lettuce leaf as your wrap.

# 15.Keto Salad Caesar special

## Ingredients

- Two-quarter pounds of chicken breast
- One tablespoon of extra virgin olive oil
- Salt and pepper to your taste preference
- Two and a half-ounce of bacon
- Seven ounces of romaine lettuce
- Your desired amount of freshly grated Parmesan cheese

dressing

- Half cup mayonnaise
- A tablespoon of mustard
- Half of a lemon or lemon juice
- Two tablespoons of cut-up filleted anchovies
- Two cloves of cut up finely garlic
- A dash of each of salt and pepper

## Instructions

- Put the temperature of your oven to 375° Fahrenheit and preheat until it reaches its temperature.

- Stir your ingredients for the dressing altogether. This being the salt and pepper to your taste preference
- Two and a half-ounce of bacon
- Seven ounces of romaine lettuce
- Your desired amount of freshly grated Parmesan cheese dressing
- Half cup mayonnaise
- A tablespoon of mustard
- Half of a lemon or lemon juice
- Take your chicken breast and set them in a pan for baking that you have greased
- Sprinkle your chicken with salt and pepper.
- Top it off with extra virgin olive oil
- Cook your chicken thoroughly for around twenty minutes until it's tender.
- Cook up the bacon until nice and crispy,
- Place your chopped lettuce on a plate along with your cut chicken and place your crumbled bacon on top.
- Enjoy your feast with the dressing you have prepared.

# 16.Roasted Sausage

## Ingredients

• Twelve Italian sausage patties

• One eggplant

• One red pepper

• One yellow pepper

• One tablespoon extra virgin olive oil

• One dry tablespoon thyme

• One tablespoon rosemary also dried

• Pinch of salt

## Instructions

• Set up your oven to cook at 400 degrees Fahrenheit.

• Slit up your sausage patties up two or three times.

• Get the sausage ready by putting on an oiled cooking sheet.

• Cut your zucchini into sizes that can fit in your mouth.

• Peel eggplant and peppers and cut into larger slices.

• Put everything that you have done so far on a baking sheet and put salt and pepper on top and then pour the oil on.

• Bake your sausage and veggies for around 35 to 40 minutes.

• When done, serve the meal.

# 17.Slow-cooked spare ribs

This is an easier recipe to make that requires just two ingredients.

## Ingredients

• Four pounds of beef pork chops

• One-third cup of pesto sauce, optionally you may add salt and pepper as well

## Instructions

• Take your slow cooker out around the time that you generally eat lunch and get your spare ribs ready to go in the cooker with pesto sauce.

• Cook on the highest setting for five to six hours.

• You can add salt and pepper if you prefer.

# 18.Shrimp Scampi

## Ingredients

• Two tablespoons olive oil from grapeseed

• Two tablespoons of store-bought Cajun seasoning

• One pound of defined-peeled fresh or frozen shrimp

• Two zucchinis that are round

• Two tablespoons of chopped up parsley

• One tablespoon of Parmesan cheese that is grated

## Directions

• Combine your grapeseed olive oil with your Cajun seasoning in a pan for frying.

• Grab your shrimp and toss it in your mixture.

• Cook your shrimp on medium to a medium-high setting.

• Heat for about three minutes on each side until both sides are pink. Add another tablespoon of grapeseed olive oil and a tablespoon of Cajun seasoning to your empty frying pan you made the shrimp in.

- Add zucchini into the mixture that you made, then put your shrimp back into the pan and cook it up for two minutes.
- The Parmesan makes a great garnish with the parsley.
- If you prefer, you can also cook up some rice as a side dish, but this will add more carbohydrates.

# 19. Pork Chop Dinner

## Ingredients

- Six brown pork loin chops
- One can of tomato sauce of your liking
- One tablespoon of olive oil
- One tablespoon brown sugar
- One large green onion
- Two tablespoons of Worcestershire sauce
- One chopped medium green pepper
- One and a half tablespoons of cider variety vinegar
- One drained four ounces can mushrooms stems
- Half teaspoon of salt
- Not cooked rice

## Instructions

- Place your brown pork chops in oil and drain them, and put in a slow cooker.
- Mix in onion with green peppers and mushrooms.
- In a bowl, put tomato sauce, brown sugar, Worcestershire sauce, vinegar, and salt together.

- Pour all this over your pork chops and let cook in the slow cooker.
- Cook your rice in your desired method and add the other items on it.

# 20.Low Carb Parm Meatballs

## Ingredients

• One pound of ground beef

• One cup grated Parmesan cheese

• One-third cup of parsley

• One egg

• Two cloves garlic that has been minced

• One tablespoon crushed red pepper

• One tablespoon Italian seasoning

• Salt and pepper to your liking

• A 24-ounce jar of your favorite brand of marinara sauce

## Directions

- First heat your oven up to 350 degrees Fahrenheit

- , Lay parchment paper along with a baking sheet.

- Put your ground beef, Parmesan cheese, crushed red pepper, Italian seasoning, garlic, egg, parsley, salt, and pepper into a bowl that you have stirred well.

- Sculpt your beef mix into inch and half-sized balls, line them along with the baking sheets.

- . Bake your meatballs in the oven until cooked through and a nice brown for about twenty minutes.

- Add your choice of marinara sauce to it.

# 21 Skillet Taco dinner

## Ingredients

- One pound beef ground up like hamburger meat
- One package of seasoning made for tacos
- Two and a half cups of water
- Seven ounces of macaroni elbows or other small shapes you enjoy pasta Four ounces of cheddar cheese that are shredded up.
- Two green onions that are cut up
- Half cup of regular sour cream
- One chopped tomato that is of average size

## Directions

- In a large skillet brown your beef using the medium to high heat until your beef is cooked all the way through.
- Remember to stir often and drain meat when needed.
- Mix in your macaroni taco mix and water.

- Reduce your heat to med-low heat after it starts to boil, then cover it for about ten minutes but uncovering here and there to mix.

- Dump onions and shredded cheese in, then place sour cream and cut up tomatoes on top and enjoy.

## 22.Creamy Tuscan Chicken

### Ingredients

- Two pounds of thin-sliced chicken without bones in it
- Two tablespoons extra-virgin olive oil
- One cup heavy cream
- Half cup chicken broth
- One teaspoon garlic powder
- One teaspoon seasoning of the Italian variety
- One cup Parmesan cheese
- One cup spinach that is chopped up
- Half a sun-dried cup tomatoes

### Directions

- Add extra virgin olive oil to a skillet and cook your chicken on the medium to a medium-high setting for approximately three to five minutes until both sides of the chicken are browned evenly.
- Take the already cooked chicken and place it to the side for later usage.

- Add chicken broth, heavy cream, garlic powder, Italian seasoning, and Parmesan cheese into a bowl and stir, using a medium setting until the combination has thickened.
- Add your tomato that is sun friend, and spinach then let simmer until the spinach has cooked.
- Add the chicken back to your skillet, then serve over if your diet allows, add brown rice, and enjoy your meal.

# 23.Crimini and kale frittata

## Ingredients

- One tablespoon of ghee

- Two garlic cloves minced up

- Eight ounces of crimini mushrooms diced up

- Two cups of de-stemmed curly kale

- Ten large eggs if you can afford it, use organic.

- Three-quarter cups of two percent milk

- A quarter cup of cheddar cheese that is grated finely

- A quarter teaspoon of regular but preferably sea salt

- A quarter teaspoon of regular black pepper

## Instructions

- get your oven ready by preheating it to 350 degrees Fahrenheit.

- Grab your ghee from the ingredients and heat over a medium to medium-high in a bigger sized pan.

- Cook up the garlic to a nice saute level for two minutes.

- Add your mushrooms and saute those for an additional five minutes.
- Add your kale as well as the crimini mushrooms and fry for another five minutes until your kale is cooked.
- Add your mushrooms and kale to a pie pan.
- Dump your cheese on top of this.
- Combine and stir fast or using a whisk the eggs and milk in a bowl.
- Dump the mixture into your pie pan.
- Bake your pie pan in the oven for around flirty five to fifty-five minutes.
- Serve while still warm and enjoy.

## 24. Low Carb Carrot Cake

A cake can still be a part of a ketogenic diet when appropriately prepared. Check out this recipe for an excellent recipe that will make your taste buds dance.

### Ingredients

### CAKE:

- One and a half cups flour from almonds
- Half cup flour from coconut
- Two teaspoons of regular baking soda
- Half of a teaspoon regular baking powder
- One and a half teaspoon of ground cinnamon
- Half teaspoon nutmeg that is ground
- A quarter teaspoon of ginger
- One cup of coconut oil
- Four eggs
- Two teaspoons extracted vanilla
- ¾ cup low carb sugar substitute
- One and a half cups packed grated zucchini

- One cup loosely packed grated carrots

- Half cup walnuts which are entirely optional

**FROSTING:**

- Sixteen ounces of plain cream cheese

- Half cup butter or margarine

- 2 cups regular powdered sweetener

- Two teaspoons of extracted vanilla

- Two tablespoons heavy style based whipping cream

**CAKE Directions**

- Put the oven on a setting of 350 degrees Fahrenheit.

- Place parchment paper along the bottom of two nine each cake pans.

- Mix the almond flour, coconut flour, baking powder, baking soda, cinnamon, nutmeg, and ginger in a bowl. Put completely to the side

- In another separate bowl, mix coconut oil, your four eggs, and vanilla extract.

- Stir in zucchini, carrots, and low-carbohydrate sweetener

- , then add your flour mix and stir until properly mixed.
- If using walnuts, stir them in as well.
- Spread batter evenly between the two cake pans. Smooth the tops evenly.
- Bake for twenty-five to thirty minutes until it is a light brown on top and cake feels firm when you touch it.
- Take out of the oven and cool.

**FROSTING:**

- Put together the cream cheese and butter or margarine using a mixer or whisk
- Add powdered sweetener and stir until quite smooth.
- Stir the vanilla extract and heavy whipping-style cream until fluffy and white.
- Add the frosting on top of the cake once it has cooled enough to frost.

## 25. Nutella Frosting With Low Carb Cupcakes

### Ingredients for the Cake

- A quarter cup of flour from coconuts
- A quarter cup of cocoa powder that is unsweetened
- 1 cup of baking sweetener of choice
- Quarter teaspoon cinnamon
- Single tbsp. of regular baking soda
- 1 tsp of regular baking powder
- One-eighth teaspoon of salt
- Two tablespoons liquified coconut oil
- Two large eggs slightly beaten
- Half teaspoon vanilla extract
- One cup zucchini finely grated

### FROSTING:

- Half cup butter you have let soften
- One ounce cream cheese also room temp softened
- One cup confectioners powdered sweetener
- Quarter cup hazelnut chocolate spread or Nutella

- Two Tablespoons heavy cream
- One teaspoon extracted vanilla
- Salt to taste

## Instructions

CAKE:

- Mix in a bowl baking soda, coconut flour, 70 percent cocoa, your choice of sweetener, cinnamon, salt, and baking powder
- Stir in coconut oil, the eggs, and extracted vanilla until well blended. Add in grated zucchini.
- Split batter between 8 cupcake mould greased.
- Cook at 350 degrees for twenty-five to thirty minutes.

## FROSTING:

- Stir butter and cream cheese with a mixer until creamy and smooth.
- Slowly beat in the powdered sweetener until mixed well.
- Combine the hazelnut chocolate spread and mix-in.

- Add in the heavy cream, vanilla extract, and salt and mix until fluffy.
- Add frosting on top of the cupcakes.

# 26. Bacon Cheddar Quiche with Cauliflower Crust

### Ingredients

CRUST:

- One head cauliflower
- A Quarter cup of regular mozzarella cheese shredded
- A Quarter cup of grated Parmesan cheese
- One egg
- Quarter teaspoon salt
- Quarter teaspoon garlic that is powdered

### FILLING:

- Eight slices of bacon that has been cooked and finely cut
- Four ounces of grated cheddar cheese
- A Quarter cup of Parmesan cheese
- Half cup of regular heavy cream
- Half cup regular faucet water
- Six eggs
- Quarter teaspoon table salt.

**Instructions**

CRUST:

- Grate up the cauliflower in a food processor finely.
- Put in covered microwavable dish and microwave for five to six minutes.
- Cool this without a cover for twelve minutes.
- Place your already cooked cauliflower into a cheesecloth and squeeze out all of the water that you can.
- Add dried cauliflower in a bowl with mozzarella cheese, Parmesan cheese, egg, salt, and garlic powder. Mix it up.
- Place the crust mix into the bottom of a pie plate.
- Bake at 425° FAHRENHEIT for about fourteen to nineteen minutes.
- Take out and set aside on a non-melting surface.

**FILLING**

- Pour bacon, Parmesan cheese, cheddar cheese into the crust.

- In a regular-sized bowl, mix-up the cream, water, eggs, and salt.

- Cook in the oven at 350°F for approximately forty to forty-five minutes or until filling is set.

- Take out and allow to cool slightly before serving.

# 27.Chicken and Shrimp Stir Fry

## Ingredients

- Two tablespoons coconut oil

- One thinly cut green onion

- Four cloves of garlic minced up

- Three tablespoons minced ginger

- One pound of fresh broccoli chopped up into florets or frozen florets

- One pound chicken boneless and skinned chicken that is cubed up.

- Quarter cup coconut aminos

- 11 drops liquid stevia

- One pound shrimp with tails that are frozen or fresh, peeled.

- Quarter teaspoon sea salt or regular salt if not available.

## Instructions

- In a large frying pan, melt the coconut oil over medium-high.

- Cook onions that you add to the pan until a translucent colour.
- Stir in the garlic and ginger and stir fry until cooked.
- Dump in the broccoli and fry for about ten to 11 more minutes.
- Add the coconut aminos and stevia.
- Then, stir in the chicken, shrimp, and salt.
- Cook until shrimp is cooked all the way through.
- Serve hot over cauliflower rice.

## 28.Korean BBQ Slow Cooker Ribs

### Ingredients

- Two pounds pork ribs

- One and a half cups BBQ sauce

- Six ounces baby carrots cut in half

- Four boiling onions peeled

- Five cloves garlic peeled

### DIRECTIONS

- Set the vegetables at the bottom of a slow cooker and add the spare ribs on top.

- Cover with the BBQ Sauce and cook on high for five to six hours.

- Salt to taste and serve hot and enjoy

# 29. BLT Chicken salad

## Ingredients

- Half a cup regular or low-fat mayo
- Three tablespoons of barbecue sauce
- Two tablespoons finely chopped onion
- One tablespoon fresh lemon squeezed or lemon juice
- One teaspoon black pepper
- Eight cups cut salad greens
- Two chopped tomatoes
- One and a half pounds skinless and without bones of chicken breasts, cooked and cubed
- Eleven bacon pieces cooked up then crumbled
- Two eggs you have pre-hard-boiled and sliced

## Instructions

- In a bowl, combine the first five ingredients and mix them well.
- Cover and refrigerate these until serving the entire meal.
- Put salad greens in a bowl.

- Add tomatoes, chicken, and bacon
- Add the boiled eggs.
- Dump on the dressing.
- Serve and enjoy

# 30.Pan-Roasted Salmon with Cherry Tomatoes

### Ingredients.

- Two cups of cherry tomatoes, cut in half
- One tablespoon regular olive oil
- Quarter teaspoon kosher or regular salt
- Quarter teaspoon black ground-up pepper

### Salmon

- Four salmon fillets
- Half a teaspoon regular or kosher salt
- Quarter teaspoon black pepper
- One tablespoon olive oil
- Two garlic cloves, minced
- Three quarters cup lower if possible sodium chicken broth

### Directions

- Heat the oven to 425 degrees Fahrenheit.

  Put the tomatoes in a foiled baking pan.

- Cover with foil, put salt and pepper on top

- Toss to coat.

- Cook until tomatoes are soft for about nine to twelve minutes making sure to stir.

- Meanwhile, coat the fillets with salt and pepper.

- In a large frying pan, heat oil over medium to high flame.

- Add fillets and cook three to four minutes on each side.

- Remove from pan.

- Add garlic to pan, cook, and stir for about a minute.

- Add broth, stirring to loosen browned bits from pan.

- Bring to a boil, cook until liquid is drained by half for one to two minutes.

- Stir in roasted tomatoes and return salmon to the pan.

- Bake until fish begins to flake with a fork, for four to seven minutes.

- Four slices pancetta

- One tablespoon regular olive oil

- One finely chopped shallot

- Three-quarter cup chopped or canned mushrooms
- Quarter teaspoon salt
- Quarter teaspoon pepper
- Four skinned and boneless chicken halves
- Half cup premade pesto

**Directions**

- Set the oven to 350 degrees Fahrenheit
- In a frying pan, cook pancetta over medium until partially cooked but not crispy, then drain on regular paper towels.
- In the same pan, heat oil over medium to high setting.
- Add shallot, stir until lightly browned for one to three minutes.
- Stir in mushrooms
- Cook them until tender for about two minutes.
- Add one-eighth teaspoon salt and one-eighth teaspoon pepper.
- Mash chicken breasts with a mallet made for meat mashing to a quarter-inch thickness.

- Spread each with two tablespoons pesto; layer with one slice pancetta and a fourth of mushroom mixture.
- Fold chicken in half and keep in place with toothpicks.
- Add the other ⅛ remaining salt and pepper.
- Transfer to a greased baking dish and cook until a thermometer states it is 165 degrees Fahrenheit, usually for thirty to thirty-five minutes.
- Get rid of toothpicks and serve.

# 31. Cajun Sirloin with mushroom

## Ingredients

- One and a quarter lbs of beef top sirloin steak
- Two tablespoons basic Cajun seasoning
- Two tablespoons extra-virgin olive oil
- Half pound sliced assorted fresh mushrooms or canned if not available
- One medium leek (white portion only), and sliced in half
- One tablespoon butter or margarine
- One teaspoon garlic that is minced up
- One and a half cups dry red wine
- One-quarter teaspoon pepper
- One-eighth teaspoon salt

## Directions

- Put the Cajun seasoning on the steak and let stand for seven minutes.
- In a skillet, cook steak in extra virgin oil over medium to high heat for seven to ten minutes on each side.

- Remove and keep heated.

- In the same pan, saute mushrooms and pour in butter or margarine until tender.

- Add garlic and cook one to two minutes longer.

- Add wine, pepper, and salt, stirring

- Bring to a boil then cook until liquid has dropped by half.

- Slice steak and serve with mushroom sauce to your pleasure.

# 32.Mexican Turkey Meatloaf

Ingredients

- Two pieces of plain white bread diced into tiny pieces
- One-third cup one percent or skim milk
- One lb lean turkey that is ground up
- Half lb chorizo
- One finely chopped sweet red pepper
- One onion cut up
- Single Pepper of the jalapeno variety
- Two beaten eggs
- Two tablespoons of cilantro
- Two cloves of minced garlic
- Two teaspoons of the spicy chili powder
- One teaspoon salt
- One teaspoon cumin ground up
- Half teaspoon of oregano
- Half teaspoon pepper
- A Quarter teaspoon of cayenne pepper spice
- Two-thirds cups of your salsa choice
- More diced up cilantro

- Hot cooked rice of the Spanish variety

## Directions

- Put together bread and milk in a bowl and allow it to settle.
- Combine your additional 14 ingredients and one-third cup salsa, thoroughly mix.
- Using foil, mould the meat mix into an oval, elongated shape.
- Grab the foil, move to an oval slow cooker.
- Along sides of the slow cooker, press edges of the foil.
- Cook while completely covered until it is included on low until it's 165 degrees.
- Grab edges of the foil and lift.
- Pour the fat into the cooker before you take the meatloaf to a platter.
- Put the rest of the salsa and cilantro on top.
- Wait ten minutes to cool down before you slice it and serve it.

# 33.Pot Roast and Asian Black Bean

## Ingredients

- One boneless beef chuck roast 4 pounds
- Half teaspoon table salt
- Half teaspoon black pepper
- One tablespoon regular olive oil
- One onion, cut into 1-inch pieces
- Three-fourths cup Asian black bean sauce
- One-fourth cup beef broth
- Half pound sliced fresh or canned mushrooms
- Eight ounces fresh snow peas, trimmed
- One tablespoon cornstarch
- One tablespoon chilled water
- Hot cooked brown rice
- Four sliced green onions

## Directions

- Dash the salt and pepper on the roast
- In a frying pan, heat oil over medium-high heat.
- Brown roast four to five minutes on each side.

- Move to a slow cooker. Add onion.
- Mix black bean sauce and broth, then dump over the roast.
- Cook, covered, on low for about five to six hours.
- Afterward, add mushrooms and snow peas and continue cooking on low until meat is tender for around a half-hour.
- Remove roast and vegetables to a serving plate, but keep it warm.
- Move cooking juices to a saucepan.
- Bring cooking juices to a boil.
- In a bowl, mix cornstarch and chilled water, then stir into cooking juices.
- Get it to a boil; cook and mix one to two minutes or until thick.
- Serve roast with hot cooked rice and sauce.
- Sprinkle on top the green onions, salt, and black pepper.

# 34.Chicken and garlic with fresh herbs

## Ingredients

- Six chicken thighs that are boneless and skinned
- Half teaspoon table salt
- Quarter teaspoon black pepper
- One tablespoon regular olive oil
- Ten peeled and cut in half garlic cloves
- Two tablespoons Brandy
- One cup chicken stock
- One teaspoon minced fresh rosemary
- Half teaspoon minced fresh thyme
- One tablespoon minced fresh chives

## Directions

- Sprinkle chicken with salt and pepper.
- In a cast-iron pan, heat oil over the medium-high setting.
- Brown chicken fully on both sides.
- Take out of the pan.

- Remove skillet from flame then add halved garlic cloves and brandy.
- Heat your flame, cook, and mix over medium settings until liquid is almost evaporated.
- Mix in the stock, rosemary, and thyme.
- Add chicken to the pan again.
- Bring to a boil, lower heat, simmer, uncovered, until a thermometer reads 170 degrees Fahrenheit,
- Sprinkle with chives.

# 35.Bacon and tomato haddock

## Ingredients

- Six chopped bacon strips

- One thinly sliced medium onion

- One minced garlic clove

- One cup panko bread crumbs

- Two chopped plum tomatoes

- Quarter cup parsley

- Two tablespoons of premium olive oil

- One tablespoon melted butter

- Five haddock fillets (Six ounces each)

- Two tablespoons freshly squeezed lemon juice

- Quarter teaspoon salt

## Directions

- In a pan, cook bacon using the medium settings mostly cooked but not too

- crisp.

- Mix garlic and onion cooking to a golden-brown colour, mix it here and there for ten to fifteen minutes.

- Take off the stove and mix the bread crumbs in as well as parsley and tomatoes.

- Set this somewhere nearby.

- Set the oven to cook to 400 degrees.

- Grease up a baking pan with oil and butter

- Put your fillets in the pan you are using

- Squeeze the lemon juice on and add a dash of salt

- Put it in the bread crumb mixture

- Cook in the oven for ten to fifteen minutes

# 36. Fortina Rolled chicken

## Ingredients

- Four ounces cream cheese

- One cup grated fontina cheese

- Six bacon strips cooked and crumbled

- Four chopped up green onions

- Quarter cup chopped Italian parsley

- Quarter cup julienned oil-packed sun-dried tomatoes, drained, cut up and patted dry

- Half teaspoon table salt

- Three-Quarter teaspoon black pepper

- One egg

- One and a half cups panko bread crumbs

- One teaspoon paprika

- Four six ounces skinned and boneless chicken breast halves

## Directions

- Heat oven to 375 degrees Fahrenheit

- In a bowl, Stir the first six ingredients

- Stir in a quarter teaspoon each salt and pepper.

- In a bowl, whisk egg, salt, and pepper.
- In another shallow bowl, put the bread crumbs with paprika.
- Carefully crush chicken breasts with a meat mallet to a quarter-inch thickness.
- Spread cheese mixture over chicken.
- Roll up chicken from a short side and secure with toothpicks.
- Dip chicken in egg, then coat with crumbs.
- Place in a foil-lined baking pan and seam side down.
- Pour oil over it.
- Bake without the top a half-hour to thirty-five minutes or until golden brown
- Let stand 5 minutes and get rid of toothpicks before serving.

# 37.Dilly BBQ Turkey

## Ingredients

- One cup plain yogurt
- Half cup lemon juice
- Third cup canola oil
- Half cup minced up parsley
- Half cup chopped green onions
- Four minced garlic cloves
- Four tablespoons fresh minced dill
- One teaspoon dried and crushed up rosemary
- One teaspoon salt
- Half teaspoon pepper
- One turkey breast (two and a half to three pounds)

## Directions

- In a bowl, put together the first ten ingredients.
- Dump half into a large resealable plastic bag and put it into the turkey.
- Close up the bag and shake vigorously to marinate.
- Cover and refrigerate overnight.
- Cover and refrigerate remaining yogurt.

- Drain and throw away marinade from Turkey.

- Grill turkey and covered, over medium-high heat while often basting with reserved marinade for one hour

- Serve hot with table salt and black pepper

# 38.Chicken Alfredo and grilled apple

## Ingredients

- Four 6 oz. boneless, skinned chicken breast halves
- Four teaspoons your fave chicken seasoning
- One large Gala apple, cut into half-inch wedges
- One tablespoon lemon juice
- Four thin slices provolone cheese
- Half cup warm Alfredo sauce
- Quarter cup blue cheese crumbled up

## Directions

- Put chicken seasoning on both sides of chicken
- In a bowl, toss together your apple wedges with lemon juice.
- Wet a paper towel with canola oil.
- Using tongs, rub on grill rack to coat lightly.
- Grill chicken, with a cover, over medium settings for five to eight minutes on each side or until a thermometer reads 165 degrees Fahrenheit.

- Grill the apple over medium heat two to three minutes on each side or until browned.

- Add chicken with provolone cheese and cook, covered, one to two minutes longer, or until cheese is melted.

- Serve chicken with Alfredo sauce, apples and put on the blue cheese.

# 39.Scallops with spinach

## Ingredients

- Four bacon strips chopped up
- Twelve sea scallops with side muscles taken out
- Two shallots, finely chopped
- Half cup white wine
- Eight cups baby spinach

## Instructions

- In a large skillet, cook bacon over medium heat until crisp and mix occasionally.
- Remove with a slotted spoon and drain on paper towels.
- Discard drippings, but keep two tablespoons.
- Wipe skillet clean.
- Pat scallops dry with paper towels.
- In the same skillet, heat one tablespoon drippings over medium to high heat and add scallops and cook until golden brown.
- Remove from pan; keep heated warm.

- Use remaining drippings in the same pan over medium-high flame.

- Add shallot, cook, and stir until tender, two to three minutes.

- Add wine and bring to a boil, stirring to loosen browned bits from pan.

- Add spinach, then cook and stir until wilted, one to two minutes.

- Stir in bacon and serve with scallops.

# 40.Baked Mushroom Chicken

## Ingredients

- Four skinned and boneless chicken breast halves
- Quarter cup basic flour
- Three tablespoons butter or margarine divided
- One cup sliced fresh mushrooms or canned
- Half cup chicken broth
- A quarter teaspoon of table or sea salt
- One-eighth teaspoon black pepper
- One-third cup shredded part-skim mozzarella cheese
- One-third cup grated Parmesan cheese
- Quarter cup sliced green onions

## Directions

- Make sure each chicken breast is flattened to a quarter-inch thickness.
- Place flour in a bowl.
- Dip chicken in flour to coat both sides; shake off the excess flour.
- In a frying pan, cook chicken in two tablespoons butter or margarine on both sides.

- Move to a greased baking dish.
- In the same pan, cook mushrooms in the leftover butter or margarine until tender.
- Add the broth, table salt, and black pepper.
- Bring to a boil; cook until liquid is brought down to about a half-cup, about five minutes.
- Spoon over chicken.
- Bake without a cover, at 375 degrees Fahrenheit until chicken is done.
- Sprinkle lightly with cheese and green onions.
- Bake until cheese is melted.
- Serve and enjoy.

•

## 41. Ketolicious vanilla sauce and Cinnamon Apples

You are not going to believe that a low carb dessert could be this delicious. This is absolutely a dream desert.

## Ingredients

- Your Desired Amount of Vanilla sauce
- Three cups of whipped heavy cream
- Half of a teaspoon extracted vanilla
- Two tablespoons butter or margarine
- A Single yolk from an egg

## Ingredients for Cinnamon apples

- Three tablespoons margarine or butter
- Three apples
- One teaspoon cinnamon that is finely ground

## Instructions

- Combine margarine or butter and vanilla in a pan with one-quarter of the whipped heavy cream
- Lightly boil using medium heat in the saucepan
- After it is lightly cooked, set it on low heat and for five minutes let it simmer
- Make sure you are stirring it consistently
- Turn the heat off and put the egg yolk in and mix it fast
- Put it in the refrigerator and coo

- The rest of the heavy whip cream whisk it in a bowl to a creamy texture
- Use the sauce that's in the fridge and fold with the whipped cream
- Next put it back in the refrigerator for a half an hour
- Peel the apples and core them
- Slice the apples thinly
- Get a frying pan and fry apples until they are a golden light brown colour
- Add cinnamon
- With the vanilla sauce recipe given below, serve the apples while they are still warm
- If you choose to do so, you may make the cream up to twenty-four hours before and keep in the fridge.

**The vanilla sauce**

**Ingredients**

- Use four lightly whipped egg yolks
- Half of a cup of sugar
- Two full cups of fat-free milk
- One teaspoon of vanilla extract

- Half of a cup of sugar

## Instructions

- Stir together in a beating fashion, the four egg yolks, and sugar until the yolk of the eggs is a light yellow colour.
- Boil the milk in a saucepan and pour over the mixture you just prepared in a stream that is thin using an electric mixer or you can whisk it if you don't have one.
- Put the combined mixture into a pan and without boiling, heat to a point where it can coat a spoon on the back
- Add the vanilla extract after taking the pan off the stovetop and stir together all ingredients
- The sauce can be used either hot or cold, depending on your preference. Remove the pan from the heat and stir in vanilla extract if you are using it.

# 42. Ketogenic Banana Waffles

If you love both bananas and waffles, then you are in luck. This is a dairy-free low carb version that is also great for those who are lactose intolerant.

## Ingredients

- A single banana that is ripened
- Five eggs
- ¾ cups of almond flour
- 3/4 cup of milk from a coconut
- A total of a single tablespoon of baking powder
- A Single teaspoon of extracted vanilla
- Coconut oil
- A Single tablespoon of powdered ground psyllium husk powder
- Single dash of salt
- A Single teaspoon of ground-up cinnamon

**Instructions**

- Combine all of your ingredients in a bowl and whisk it.

- Next, let the mixture sit for half n hour.

- Use either a frying pan or if you have one, a waffle-making device, and use coconut oil to coat the bottom.

- Make in a waffle maker in a frying pan with coconut oil and or butter.

- Serve with hazelnut spread or whipped coconut cream and some fresh berries, or have them with melted butter.

# 43.Low-carb chocolate and peanut squares

Chocolate and peanut butter go together like dogs and a chew bone.

## Ingredients

- Single dash of salt
- Use 3.5 ounces of cocoa that has at a minimum of 70 cocoa solids
- A Single teaspoon of ground licorice
- 4 tablespoons of coconut oil
- ¼ cup of creamy peanut butter
- ½ tablespoon of extracted vanilla
- Dash of cinnamon
- 1.5 ounces of hazelnuts or salted peanuts

## Instructions

- Heat until it melts, the coconut oil and chocolate in a microwave oven.

- Get a glass bowl and put it on top of a pot of steaming water.

- It's essential that the water doesn't touch the bowl because the chocolate will further melt because of the steaming heat coming off the boiling water.

- Before going on to the next step, put aside the chocolate that you melted too cool for a little bit before you go to the next instruction.

- Excluding the nuts, place the rest of the ingredients in a bowl, and mix them into a blended texture.

- Dump the batter that you mixed together into a baking dish that you have greased that is of smaller size and line it with parchment paper.

- The batter that you put aside earlier, when it is finally set, cut it into squares that are no bigger than an inch in diameter.

- Place the nuts that are chopped up on top of the recipe.

- You can either put it in the freezer or the refrigerator, depending on your preference of how long you want to wait for it to set completely.

# 44.Zero-bread Low Carb Sandwich for Breakfast

This innovative sandwich is absolutely delicious with incredible cheese, eggs, and ham together to create a genuinely delectable low carb sandwich, excluding the bread.

## Ingredients

- 2 tablespoons of margarine or butter
- 4 eggs
- Dashes of salt and pepper
- A single ounce of deli ham and pastrami
- 2 ounces of provolone cheese or cheddar cheese that is thickly sliced
- 4 drops of Worcestershire sauce

## Instructions

- Place butter in a bigger size skillet and put it on medium heat.
- Cook the five eggs over-easy on both sides.

- Add your desired amount of pepper and salt to your liking.
- As the base of your sandwich, you are going to want to use the egg.
- Add the ham and pastrami after the egg then place the cheese. Add another egg to the top of the sandwich.
- Keep it in the pan on a lower heat setting to melt the cheese and meat.
- Add 4 drops of Worcestershire sauce, and eat or serve immediately.
- If you so choose, French Dijon mustard goes well on top of the sandwich. You can also choose to use bacon instead of ham if you like as well.

---

# 45. Keto cheese and Mushroom frittata

Some people call this the Italian style omelet and as frittatas are simple to make and you can enjoy them as a meal any time of the day.

## Ingredients

- Get a Frittata
- 1 pound fresh or canned mushrooms
- Five ounces of margarine or butter
- 8 scallions
- A Single tablespoon of parsley
- ¾ teaspoon of black pepper
- 10 eggs
- One tablespoon white wine vinegar
- 10 ounces of your choice of shredded cheese
- Single-cup of mayo
- 5 ounces of lettuce or leafy greens
- Vinaigrette dressing
- 4 tablespoons of olive oil

- ¾ teaspoon of salt

## Instructions

- Prepare to cook your meal by putting the settings on 350 degrees Fahrenheit until it reaches that temperature.

- Get out the vinaigrette and put it to the side

- cut up your fresh mushrooms or open up a can of mushrooms that are already sliced.

- Heat your mushrooms on a medium-high setting using butter until it is a golden colour but don't use all the butter yet.

- Lower the temperature a little bit and use the leftover butter for later.

- cut up your scallions and combine them with the mushrooms you have already fried

- Mixing parsley and salt and pepper in a separate bowl, combine the mayo, cheese, and eggs.

- Grease up a baking dish and combine the mushrooms and scallions and dump everything else, including the cheese into the baking dish and cook for between 35 to 40 minutes, depending on when the frittata browns and the eggs are fully cooked.

- When it's done, make sure to let it cool down for a few minutes and serve it with a side of lettuce or leafy greens and the vinaigrette.

# 46. Egg and mackerel plate

A quick and easy keto meal that will keep you satiated for hours. Barely any cooking required, perfect for those busy weekdays or when you don't feel like getting busy in the kitchen.

## Ingredients

- Four eggs
- Two tablespoon butter for frying
- Eight ounces canned mackerel in tomato sauce
- Two ounces lettuce
- Half-red onion
- Quarter cup olive oil
- salt and pepper

## Instructions

- Cook the eggs in butter, sunny side up or over easy.
- Put lettuce, thin slices of red onion and mackerel on a plate together with the eggs

- Season for flavor with salt and pepper.

- Drizzle olive oil over the salad and serve.

## 47. Low Carb or Ketogenic Gravy With Biscuits

Gravy and biscuits are comforting food and make you feel full. You can still have some carbs on a low-carb diet, as mentioned before, and this is one that you can have safely while on your diet.

### Ingredients

- 4 Biscuits
- 1 cup of flour created from almonds
- ¼ teaspoon of regular or sea salt
- A single teaspoon of regular baking powder
- 4 whites from eggs
- 2 tablespoon of cold butter
- You can either have one teaspoon of any seasoning that you like or use garlic powder.
- A single teaspoon of a can of spray coconut oil
- Gravy instructions below
- 12 ounces of pork sausage
- 1 cup of coconut cream cheese

- A single cup of chicken broth

- Pepper and salt

**Instructions**

**The Biscuits**

- Set your oven to 400 degrees Fahrenheit. Get a cookie sheet and spray it down with coconut spray made of coconut oil.

- Whisk the egg whites that you have until they are very firm and have a fluffy like texture.

- Get a separate bowl to combine the almond flour and baking powder.

- Next, put in cold butter and add the salt level that you prefer. It's important that the butter is very cold, or the biscuits won't turn out the correct texture.

- Next, get the dry mixture folded into the egg whites.

- Get a spoon and take the dough and place each biscuit individually on the tray that you are cooking on.

- Put your ingredients in the oven for approximately 11 to 15 minutes until it is the texture that you desire.

**Making the Gravy**

- Using your pork sausage, cook it in a skillet using medium heat for approximately 5 to 7 minutes on high while you stir it consistently.

- Make sure to gradually add the coconut cream cheese and chicken broth and cook until your ingredients are at a simmering level and begin to thicken up.

- Don't forget to keep stirring as much as possible until you have a creamy texture.

- Change the heat settings to low-medium and let it cook for two more minutes while you are consistently stirring.

- Add salt and pepper to your mix as much as you prefer.

- Cut your biscuits into two pieces for each biscuit.

- Put the two halves of a whole biscuit on a plate with about a third of a cup of the gravy.

- Another thing you can do if you enjoy cheese is to put Parmesan on the dough before the biscuits go into the oven for a different type of flavor.

## 48. Low-carb eggplant hash with eggs

if you are a fan of potato hash, then you must try the low carb version. It is super simple to make, and most people love this low carb variety of breakfast.

### Ingredients

- Get one yellow onion and dice it up as finely as possible
- 2 tablespoons of olive oil
- Three-quarters of a pound of cubed halloumi cheese,
- Cut up two eggplants
- Pepper and salt
- Four eggs
- Two tablespoons of butter

### Instructions

- Start recipe out by putting a pan on medium heat and Fry the onion until it is soft.

- . Next, combine the eggplant and halloumi cheese and in a frying pan, cook it until the ingredients are a golden brown.
- Add your pepper and salt to your desired level
- You can cook the eggs however you like them. Make sure you're using a different pan.
- If you so desire, you may add in additional ingredients of Worcester sauce to add a little bit of extra flavor. This part is optional, however.

# 49.Low Carb frittata decorated with spinach

This delightful dish is amazingly easy to prepare. Sausage, spinach, eggs, or bacon, and your choice of veggies are put together to create a feast for your tummy.

## Ingredients

- Six ounces of cut up bacon
- Two tablespoons of margarine or butter
- 9 ounces of extremely fresh spinach
- Eight eggs
- A single cup of heavy cream that is whipped
- Six ounces of shredded cheese of your choice
- Dashes of pepper and salt to add flavor

## Instructions

- Begin by getting the oven preheated to 350 degrees.
- Spray or Grease a 9x9 cooking dish
- Use a frying pan for cooking the bacon in butter or margarine

- Do this until crispy

- When done, add the spinach until it is a wilted type of texture.

- Set aside the pan when done after removing from the oven top

- Mix the heavy whipping cream and the right eggs and put it into the dish for baking.

- Put the spinach, cheese, and bacon at the top level of the meal

- Place the pan in the middle section of the oven. Move the metal trays if possible

- Cook thoroughly for a half hour or until you see the middle is cooked by placing a toothpick in to tell, and it's a golden-brown color on top.

- Add salt and pepper to your liking and serve while hot and enjoy.

# 50.Muffin and Egg Delight

This is a straightforward and time-saving option for a low carb diet. It can be reheated with ease and is perfect for taking with you to work or sending the muffins to school for the kids.

## Ingredients

- Two diced up scallions
- Six ounces of salami or bacon, whichever you prefer
- Dozen eggs
- An optional choice is to add two tablespoons of green or red pesto
- Dashes of salt and pepper
- Seven ounces of your choice of finely shredded cheese.

## Instructions

- Begin by setting the oven to cook at a temperature of three hundred and fifty degrees Fahrenheit.

- If you have a muffin tin, grease it or use baking cups if you prefer.
- Put your scallions at the very bottom of the tin.
- Combine a dozen eggs with the pesto if you decide to add that
- Add a dash of salt and pepper as well as the cheese and stir profoundly until creamy with no lumps.
- Put the mixed up batter above the scallions
- Depending on the size of your muffin tins, you will bake it for approximately fifteen to twenty minutes.

# FINAL WORDS

Thank you again for purchasing this book!

We really hope this book is able to help you.

The next step is for you to **join our email newsletter** to receive updates on any upcoming new book releases or promotions. You can sign-up for free and as a bonus, you will also receive our "*7 Fitness Mistakes You Don't Know You're Making*" book! This bonus book breaks down many of the most common fitness mistakes and will demystify many of the complexities and science of getting into shape. Having all this fitness knowledge and science organized into an actionable step-by-step book will help you get started in the right direction in your fitness journey! To join our free email newsletter and grab your free book, please visit the link and signup: **www.effingopublishing.com/gift**

Finally, if you enjoyed this book, then we would like to ask you for a favor, would you be kind enough to leave a review for this book? It would be greatly appreciated! Thank you and good luck in your journey!

# About the Co-Author

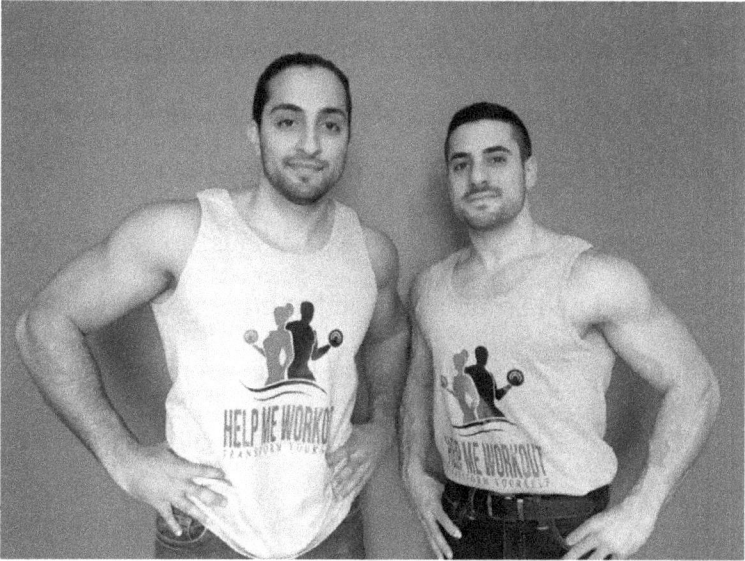

Our name is Alex & George Kaplo; we're both certified personal trainers from Montreal, Canada. Will start off by saying we are not the biggest guys you will ever meet and this has never really been our goal. In fact, we started working out to overcome our biggest insecurity when we were younger, which was our self-confidence. You may be going through some challenges right now, or you may simply want to get fit, and we can certainly relate.

For us personally, we always kind were interested in the health & fitness world and wanted to gain some muscle due to the numerous bullying in our teenage years. We figured we can do something about how our body looks like. This was the beginning of our transformation journey. We had no idea where to start, but we both just got started. We felt worried and afraid at times that other people would make fun of us for doing the exercises the wrong way. We always wished we had a friend to guide us and who could just show us the ropes.

After a lot of work, studying and countless trial and errors. Some people began to notice how we were both getting more fit and how we were starting to form a keen interest in the topic. This led many friends and new faces to come to us and ask us for fitness advice. At first, it seemed odd when people asked us to help them get in shape. But what kept us going is when they started to see changes in their own body and told us it's the first time that they saw real results! From there, more people kept coming to us, and it made both of us realize after so much reading and studying in this field that it did help us but it also allowed us to help others. To date, we have coached and trained numerous clients who have achieved some pretty amazing results.

Today, both of us own & operate this publishing business, where we bring passionate and expert authors to write about health and fitness topics. We also run an online fitness business and we would love to connect with you by inviting you to visit the website on the following page and signing up to our e-mail newsletter (you will even get a free book).

Last but not least, if you are in the position we were once in and you want some guidance, don't hesitate and ask... will be there to help you out!

Your coaches,

**Alex & George Kaplo**

# Download another book for Free

We want to thank you for purchasing this book and offer you another book (just as long and valuable as this book), "Health & Fitness Mistakes You Don't Know You're Making", completely free.

Visit the link below to signup and receive it:

www.effingopublishing.com/gift

In this book, we will break down the most common health & fitness mistakes, you are probably committing right now, and will reveal how you can easily get in the best shape of your life!

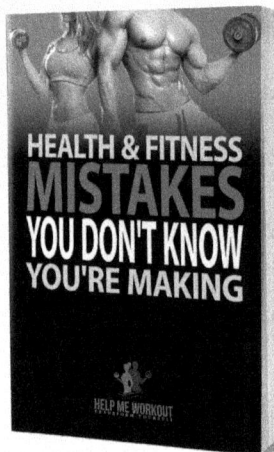

In addition to this valuable gift, you will also have an opportunity to get our new books for free, enter giveaways, and receive other valuable emails from us. Again, visit the link to sign up:

www.effingopublishing.com/gift

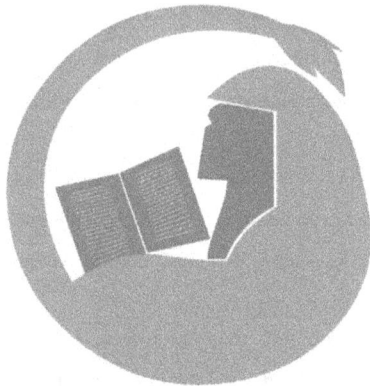

**EFFINGO**
Publishing

For more great books visit:

EffingoPublishing.com

www.ingramcontent.com/pod-product-compliance
Lightning Source LLC
Chambersburg PA
CBHW050727030426
42336CB00012B/1439